This Journal Belongs To:

Name _____

Address_____

_____

Phone _____

Email _____

We hope you have enjoyed using this book.
It would really help us a lot if you would
take a moment to leave a review.
Many thanks!

Appreciation Notebooks

Looking for an fun thank you gift?
Check out our book catalog at:

amazon.com/author/appreciationnotebooks

Made in the USA
Monee, IL
10 March 2023

29595716R10063